Discover How You Can Turn Activity Into Energy

Discover How You Can Turn Activity Into Energy

Robert H. Schuller

Harvest House Publishers
Irvine, California 92714

DISCOVER HOW YOU CAN TURN ACTIVITY INTO ENERGY

Copyright © 1978 by Robert H. Schuller
ISBN: 0-89081-135-0

CONTENTS

1

Recycle Your Energy

The Bible is filled with many statements indicating that our relationship to God vitally affects our human energy output. The prophet Isaiah wrote:

"They that wait upon the Lord shall renew their strength. They shall mount up with wings as eagles; they shall run and not be weary; and they shall walk and not faint" (Isaiah 40:31)

St. Paul wrote to the people in Ephesus that he was praying for them,

"That out of his glorious, unlimited resources He will give you the mighty inner strengthening of his Holy Spirit" (Ephesians 3:16)

Emerson wrote, "The world belongs to the energetic." And Sir Thomas Buxton agreed when he said, "The longer I live, the more deeply I am convinced that what makes the difference between one man and another, the great and the insignificant, is energy; that invincible determination, a purpose that once formed, nothing can take away. This energetic quality will do anything that is meant by God to be done in this world, and no talent, no training, no opportunity, no circumstance will make any man a man without it."

Obviously, there is a difference in energy levels from one person to another. The question is "Why?" What makes the difference? Can anyone learn to live on a more dynamic energetic level?

I want to share with you some principles on how to recycle your energy so that you'll never really suffer from real fatigue again. The honest truth is that hard work does not produce fatigue, and real rest does not heal fatigue. Psychological observations and studies show that nine tenths of all fatigue among sedentary people is psychological and emotional. And that means it is also theological, because you cannot divide psychology from theology. You cannot take the human soul and slice it into sections and say, "This section is the brain, this section is the emotion, this section is the soul, and this section is the mind that needs to be healed by psychiatry." The true person is a whole human being, and sectionalism is improper when we think of healing humans. If it is a psychological problem then it is a theological problem.

I am blessed by God with tremendous energy and have been all my life. But I don't think that I genetically have more energy than other people. My testimony to you is this very simple thing: *"In Him* (meaning in God and in Christ) *we live,* (that means we are really alive) *and move,* (instead of sitting down and slouching and sleeping lazily) *and have our being."* (Acts 17:28) The truth is, God is the cosmic source of all spiritual energy. And when we are close to God and in tune with Him, we tap the source of energy.

What I must say at the outset of this message is quite simple: Some people are tired because they're afraid they're going to get tired. And because they're afraid they're going to get tired, they don't spend their energy because they want to save it. And because they're not spending it and because they're saving it, they're constantly fatigued. If you don't have energy, the best way to get it is to give it out.

When I woke up this morning, it was still black outdoors. I had no idea what time it was. Then I heard our clock and I knew it was 5:00 a.m. "Boy, I'm still tired," I thought. "I'm still tired, and I know I won't go back to sleep now." (What a negative thought! If you think you won't go back to sleep, naturally you won't go back to sleep!) So I had a battle with myself on the pillow. And then I thought, "If I want energy, the best way to get it is not to spend another sixty minutes in bed. The best way to get it is to jump out of bed, get my running suit on and take a long run."

Actually, I was too tired to run, which was only proof of the fact that that was exactly what I had to do. So I jumped out of bed, got my running suit on and started running off into the hills. Everything went fine until in the utter darkness I turned down the wrong road, and for the first time, I got lost while running.

But I kept running and when I reached

a deadend, I turned around. It was
starting to get light and soon I recognized
some landmarks. Before long, I found

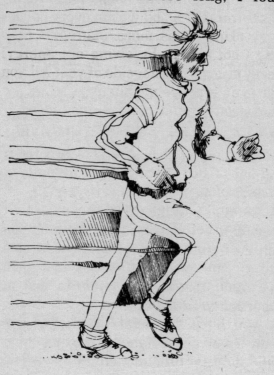

myself at my front gate—exactly 65 minutes after I started my uninterrupted run. When I got in the house and into my hot shower, the blood was in every corner of my skin. I was more energetic than ever! I got energy by giving out energy! Energy is right there inside of you! All you have to do is prime the pump.

Let me give it to you in one sentence:

WHAT YOU GET IS WHAT YOU GIVE!

You can turn it around and it still holds true:

WHAT YOU GIVE IS WHAT YOU
WILL GET!

Now that is a universal principle. If you want love from people, you have to give love. And the love that you get in return from other people is going to be in proportion to what you give.

If you have financial problems, give money away to somebody who is doing something beautiful for God. Money given is like a seed planted—it will come back to you with an increase. *"And the measure you give will be the measure you get"* (Matthew 7:2).

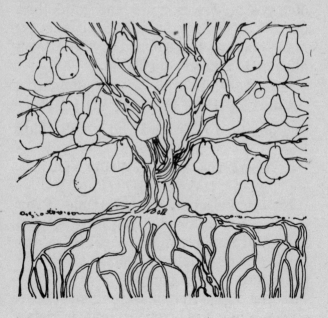

It's true for love. It's true for your money. It's true with your job. And it's true for human energy. What you give is what you will get! I call it recycled energy.

2

Energy Is a
Matter of Attitude

Several years ago, I was in Miami, Florida, to deliver a lecture at a large convention. Earlier on the program was a major address by one of the most powerful senators in the United States. Everyone would recognize his name, for it is almost a household word. I arrived early to hear his speech, and then went up to him to thank him, for it was a great speech.

I was so impressed with this man's tremendous energy. He was in his early 60's at that time, and not too long before he had discovered he had cancer. But he bounded up that stage with energy, and he spoke for 55 minutes with energy.

As I thanked him for his talk, he took hold of my arm and with misty eyes said,

"You'll never know what your Hour of Power ministry has done for me and for the rest of us in Washington, D.C." And that touched me very humbly and beautifully.

As we talked, I was impressed with the fact that energy is not a matter of age—it is a matter of attitude! It's not a matter of general health, because I see people who have had major surgery and are battling cancer, and they have loads of energy. What is the key? It's attitude! And the secret to an energetic attitude is in the reality of this verse:

"In Him we live, and move, and have our being" (Acts 17:28).

Do you need energy? Give it out and you'll get it back. Put out energy and you'll end up with more energy than you gave out. It's really true!

Now if it's true on an organic level, it is also true on the spiritual level. If you need more energy it probably means you need more faith in God. Because if you have a closer relationship with God, you'll be dreaming great dreams and attempting great things. Anybody who loves and moves in the will of God is going to be a high-energy person. *"For it is God who is at work within you, giving you the will and the power to achieve His purpose"* (See Philippians 2:13).

If you aren't energetic enough on the job, for instance, probably you're not giving your job enough. You're probably checking in as late as you can, checking out as quickly as you can and doing as little on the job as you can possibly get by with. Well, obviously in that kind of a situation you're not going to be enthused. *And enthusiasm is energy!* The word enthusiasm is made up of *en-theos*—in God.

Is Friday the best day of your week? Do

you start getting a little energy on Friday evening, more energy on Saturday and a lot of kick and get up and go on Saturday night? And on Sunday you've got quite a bit of it left, but on Monday morning when you have to go back to work, do you feel tired again?

"In Him we live, and move, and have our being." What it means is that you have to bring Christ into your life and apply Christ in your job so that you turn your job into a ministry.

Do you need energy? Do you want to recycle it? Give it out! It'll come back! Begin by making sure that you are in a close relationship with God and yourself.

Is there some secret sin in your life? If so, there will be guilt, and this guilt will block the flow of real power and energy.

Real power comes electrically through positive and negative wires. Let me say, the same is true spiritually. If you want dynamic energy, you have to be in the will of God. If you want to be in the will of God, you have to have the positive and the negative wires together. That means you have to have the power to say "no" to something that is wrong.

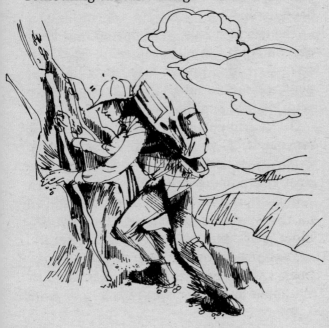

Recently I was asked to attend a board meeting at another corporation of which I am not a member of the board. The meeting was with a couple of high-powered realtors, a landowner and the landowner's lawyer. I wasn't in the meeting three minutes when the lawyer became very upset about something. I was shocked. I could tell that in that kind of a mental climate there were such negative vibrations that if I stayed around I'd be fatigued in ten minutes, and I didn't want to waste my energy. I think I said something to this effect: "When you are able to address yourselves in positive terms and with enthusiasm in a calm and reflective mind, I will be happy to return and rejoin the assembly." And with that I made a hasty exit. I could feel fatigue hanging in the room because of the negative vibrations from the cantankerous, negative-thinking lawyer.

I came back into the room a minute

later to find the lawyer storming out. (Miracles do happen!) But as soon as he got out, the quibbling and the quarrelling started again. So I suggested something which I hoped would be positive bait—and it was. They all got talking about the project that brought them together. And as they started talking about the project, they started dreaming. And as they dreamed, they got excited. And as they got excited, they got more enthusiastic. And when they started putting their ideas out, energy came back, and it was just fantastic to see the transformation that took place in that room!

Do you want energy? Power comes through the positive and the negative wires. The negative is to pull away from anything that would produce anxiety, fears, anger or guilt. The positive is drawn to anything that would produce the power to dream dreams and to get involved in projects and get excited.

There are people who use an enormous amount of energy to resist God's Holy Spirit when He tries to move into their lives. And what happens? *God stays out and they stay tired.* It's that simple.

Let me sum up, so far, with this sentence:

GREAT ACTIVITY IS NOT CAUSED
BY GREAT ENERGY,
BUT GREAT ACTIVITY PRODUCES
GREAT ENERGY.

What you give is what you get, and what you get is what you'll give. If you want the energy of God in your life, give your life to God and give your life to Jesus Christ. He'll come in and you'll be in tune with an infinite cosmic source of unending, unlimited energy that will recycle itself as you do His happy work.

3

More Energy for Better Living

There is no doubt about it—your relationship with God is a vital factor in your own human energy level.

Sometime ago a friend of ours, Don Sutton, the ace Los Angeles Dodger pitcher, was here and told us how every professional athlete looks for the edge. "Because," he said, "to really be a great success all you have to do is be just a little better than everybody else. It's that simple. All you need is the edge on the competition." "And," he said, "Jesus Christ gives me the winner's edge!" And He does, because God produces that dynamic flow of energy.

St. Paul I think was teaching this when he said, "*I can do all things through Christ who strengthens me*" (See Philippians 4:13). "In God we live and move and have our being" (Acts 17:28). "The Lord is my strength and my song, and He has become my salvation" (Exodus 15:2).

Physical energy, of course, is a matter of keeping your body in good tone, good tune, exercising right and eating right.

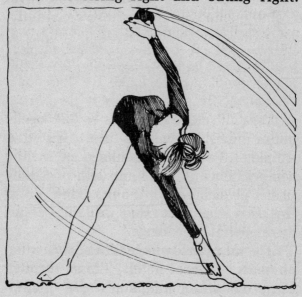

But it requires not only physical exercise, it must also have spiritual exercise. Because if a person is healthy he's a whole person. So your relationship with God definitely affects your energy level. It gives you that extra edge.

I can explain how it works. If you have a relationship with God, you're constantly excited. Excitement is a dynamic, natural energy. You say to me, "Yes, Dr. Schuller, but what about the problems?" And that's what's so exciting!

Possibility thinking is not a pollyanna philosophy that ignores the reality of problems. Possibility thinking says that every problem is pregnant with possibilities. Problems turn me on! I don't think anything would be more dull or boring than if I had no problems!

I said to a group of friends recently at a banquet in a local hotel, "I'm so excited because today I am facing the biggest problem I've ever faced in my ministry. And that really turns me on!" The problem we have in our ministry is that our sanctuary is so small that we have people standing in the aisles and in the back. And it happens every Sunday. We have what we call a growth-restricting problem. But do you know what? This problem makes me excited, *because every problem is an opportunity.* It's an opportunity for us to think bigger and reach higher. I don't believe we would ever grow unless God pushed us into it.

Robert Ardrey put it this way, "Every human being has three deep needs—the need for identity, the need for security and the need for stimulation." Now these three deep inner needs oftentimes conflict with each other. If I were to submit a test to you and say, "What is your deepest need—stimulation, security or identity?" Most people would opt for security. In other words, they want to be sure they are secure, physically and emotionally, in their interpersonal relations, in their jobs and in their finances. Security is the number one thing they're after.

But here's the problem: The road that's marked "Security" is a cul-de-sac that ends with one big sign that says, "Boredom." If you achieve ultimate security, you will achieve ultimate boredom. The

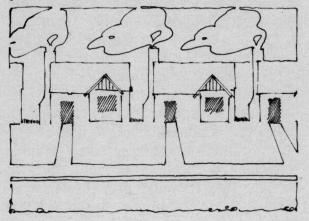

only way to escape from boredom is to expose yourself to the stimulation of some risk, some adventure or some mountain.

I've discovered in my life that possibility thinking turns me on with energy. Why? Because it helps me to escape from the road of security and commits me to the road of stimulation!

Let me illustrate very graphically about the biggest problem I have ever faced in my life. When my wife and I came to start our church twenty years ago, we had a dream of a church of 6,000 members. We thought it would take that many people to support the program, and to minister to the needs of all the people here who are hurting. It would take that many people to teach the Sunday School, to call on the sick in the hospital and to run a 24-hour telephone counselling service. And we thought that it would probably take us forty years to build up a church of 6,000 members, and so we had a plan. We planned to win 150 members a year, and in forty years, by the time I was 68, we would have 6,000 members. Then we would probably retire, leaving behind a great work that would continue to be a throbbing heart of love in the heart of this county. We thought that would make our life worthwhile.

So that was our dream. I did not, at that time, know the Alfred North Whitehead principle, which says: "Great dreams of great dreamers are never fulfilled, they are always transcended." I didn't know at that time that great dreams of great dreamers are God's dreams. And I didn't realize that God is always dreaming much bigger than I am. Because I want to play it safe, I want the stimulation, but I want to be secure, too. So I don't allow myself to dream so big that it really becomes reckless. I keep my dreams smaller, now knowing that God's dreams are always bigger. And what's happened after twenty years? We have succeeded! And what is success? When you succeed, you don't eliminate problems, you inherit bigger ones!

We had a master plan when we came to this church. We called for a sanctuary to seat nearly 2,000 people and that would handle 6,000 members running multiple services. A year ago we could see the growth curve and we made growth projections. But I turned my back on it because the only solution to that problem was to build a bigger auditorium, and I frankly didn't want to build any more buildings. I'm 48 years old, and it seems like I've been building buildings for twenty years. Not only that, but I happen to love this sanctuary. I worked on it with Richard Neutra, who is now deceased, and our sanctuary and tower are the world's finest walk-in, drive-in church.

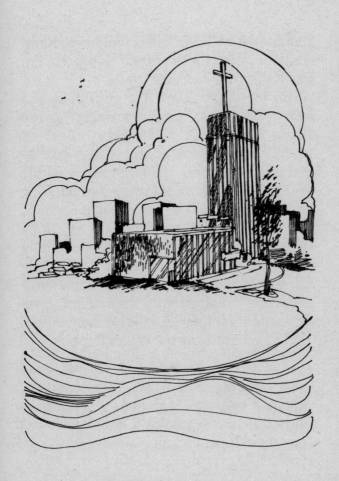

Someday it will be a historical monument. And Richard Neutra said this was the finest thing he had ever done.

Did you know that this church is the only church that is photographed in the Soviet Union? In their book of great architecture of our century, they had to include a church. It is internationally great. So I can't get interested in building buildings unless they are excellent.

I was taught a principle at Hope College, and that is, "Don't do something great; too many people already are. Only do something that excels." Excellence produces excitement. Excitement produces energy. Energy creates momentum. And momentum makes things happen!

A year ago I could see we needed a new building, and I didn't want to think about it because of the costs. I knew we didn't have the money. I was a classical negative thinker.

Well, I finally tackled the problem. The church board has unanimously agreed that we're going to solve this problem somehow. We are consulting at the present time with three of the greatest architects alive in the world today. All three are interested in the prospect of designing this new auditorium, which will be on the lawn north of our tower. It will be so beautiful that it will be an experience for people to worship there 100 years from now. It will make it possible for us to reach unchurched people in our territory and in our community.

Every morning since the first of January, 1975, I have been in the pulpit, and I can tell you, there hasn't been a Sunday when I haven't seen people turn and leave because it got too cold for them outdoors, or they were too tired to stand up in the aisle. I'm only 48, and I'm expecting to be here at least twenty more years. So finally we've decided we're going to build the building. All we need, we conclude, is $5 million. And we only have a couple hundred thousand dollars right now.

But that isn't the big problem. If I had cancer of the brain, then that would be a problem. But I'd like to make an announcement: We are going to be receiving a gift of $1 million! Isn't that great? Now I must hasten to say at this point, I don't know who is going to give it yet. But it's coming! I can feel it! Because I feel the problem so heavily. *And every time you've got a big problem, you're on the edge of a miracle!*

Nineteen years ago I stood on the sticky tar paper roof of the snack bar of the Orange Drive-In Theatre, and I said, "We are going to build a Tower of Hope. It will cost about $1 million or more, and it's coming. I don't know where it's coming from, but it's coming. And when we get it, it's going to be filled with people praying for people every minute of every hour of every day and night. We don't have any money, but God isn't poor. And He waits to pour out His abundance, but He doesn't give His riches to small-thinking people. He only gives it to those who believe big, and Lord, am I believing big!''

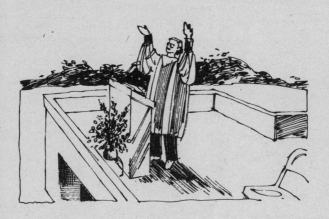

4

The Bigger the Problem, The Bigger the Miracle!

Great things are going to happen in your life as you tap into God's resource of energy! Great miracles are going to happen. I can't tell you how, but I can affirm to you with confidence that it is going to happen!

When you think this way you become energized because, you see, some people are fatigued because they don't dream any dreams. They don't dream any dreams because they want to play it safe. They don't want to get involved. They don't want to take chances. They don't want to run the risk of failure. They'd be so terribly embarrassed if later on they had to admit they were wrong. And so rather than think big and talk big, they play it safe and boy, are they dull! You will never find possibility thinkers boring,

I'll tell you that! Some people are dead, lacking energy, because they don't dream great dreams.

Then there are those that draw close enough to God until God reveals His dreams, but then they don't dare to make the decision to do anything about it. And procrastination produces fatigue. Inde-

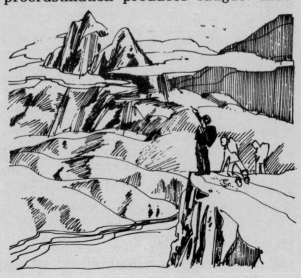

cision is the most tiring thing you could experience emotionally.

The bigger the problem, the bigger the miracle. And I don't know how God is going to use me in it, but when you're standing on the edge of something great, how can you have more energy for better living? First, find a problem of your own or a problem that somebody else has. Look for a problem that seems to be unsolvable. If you can, try to find a problem that from a human standpoint would take a miracle to get it out of the way. Then begin to pray, "Oh God, I want to thank you for this problem. Great good can come out of it. Oh God, I want to thank you for what's impossible with men is possible with you. I want to thank you for the miracles you are preparing. Oh God, I want to thank you for the faith you're giving to me now."

Pray, seek God's guidance and what's

going to happen? You'll get a dream to pursue. I have a dream to build this great new church, so that our ministry can go on and on and grow for the next twenty years. Find a dream. Once you've got that dream and you know it's God's dream for your life, then be daring. Dare to say it. Let the redeemed of the Lord say so. Announce to the whole world that it's going to happen. That is faith in action!

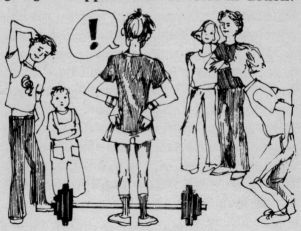

And it'll prove to people that you're not afraid of being embarrassed by failure as much as you are of being afraid of thinking too small, not having enough faith, to do something great for God.

Dream, then have nerve and be daring. And then make the decision. Let me tell you, fatigue is produced in many lives because they have no dreams; they're not excited about anything. They're not excited about anything because they cautiously try to avoid their problems and the problems of other people, because they don't want to get involved, and they don't want to make the sacrifices, and they don't want to be unselfish, and they don't want to give. So they play it safe, they ride the security road and they land up with a meaningless life. And when they die, who cares? "Only one life will soon be passed. Only what's done for Christ will last."

Some people are fatigued because they don't have any dreams, and they don't have any dreams because they avoid problems. And others have dreams, but they don't make a decision to give it all they've got. Indecision is the great fatigue producer. Make the decision to give it all you've got, and you will be astounded at the energy that will come out of you.

William James said, "You have enormous untapped powers that you probably will never tap, because most people never run far enough on their first wind to ever find out they've got a second."

I've discovered the secret to tapping enormous resources of energy in my relationship with Jesus Christ. I believe that He strengthens me, in the inner mind, through the Holy Spirit. St. Paul said, *"I can do all things through Christ who strengthens me"* (See Philippians

4:13). Literally, physically, He does!

Become an authentic Christian today. Invite Jesus Christ to be your Savior, your God and your friend. And wow! What power and energy you will discover for your life!

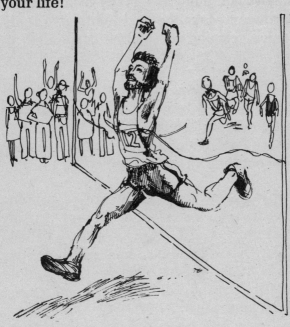

THOUGHTS, INSIGHTS

THOUGHTS, INSIGHTS